Satan's Advice for the New Parent

Satan's Advice for the New Parent

Edited by,

Aleister Lovecraft

© 2015 Aleister Lovecraft, Esq.

Cover and interior illustrations modified by the editor from public domain images obtained from the Flickr stream of the British Library.

ISBN-13: 978-1508786177
ISBN-10: 1508786178

Disclaimer: Satan is not a medical doctor. This book contains only opinions of the Prince of Darkness and should not be construed as medical advice. Please see your healthcare provider for answers to your health-related questions.

Do not reproduce any portion of this book without permission, other than for brief excerpts used for review purposes.

If you enjoyed this book, **please leave a review** where you bought it. Satan will be most pleased.

Stop by the blog at **satansadvice.tumblr.com**.

Table of Contents

Introductions 1

    Editor's Introduction 2

    Satan's Introduction 8

The One Thing 10

Part I: Pregnancy, Birth & Infancy 15

    Pregnancy 16

    Birth 20

    How to Deal with Your Newborn 25

    Sleeping 31

    Feeding 36

    Diapers 44

    Illness 48

    Discipline of Infants 51

    Adults without Children 57

    Taking Time Off Work 61

    Divorce Warning 67

Part II: Toddlers 70
Toddlers 71
Discipline of Toddlers 72
The "Playdate" 76
Toilet Training 80
What Other Parents Think 84
Cell Phones 89
Is My Child Evil? 91
Part III: Concluding Thoughts 95

To Life.

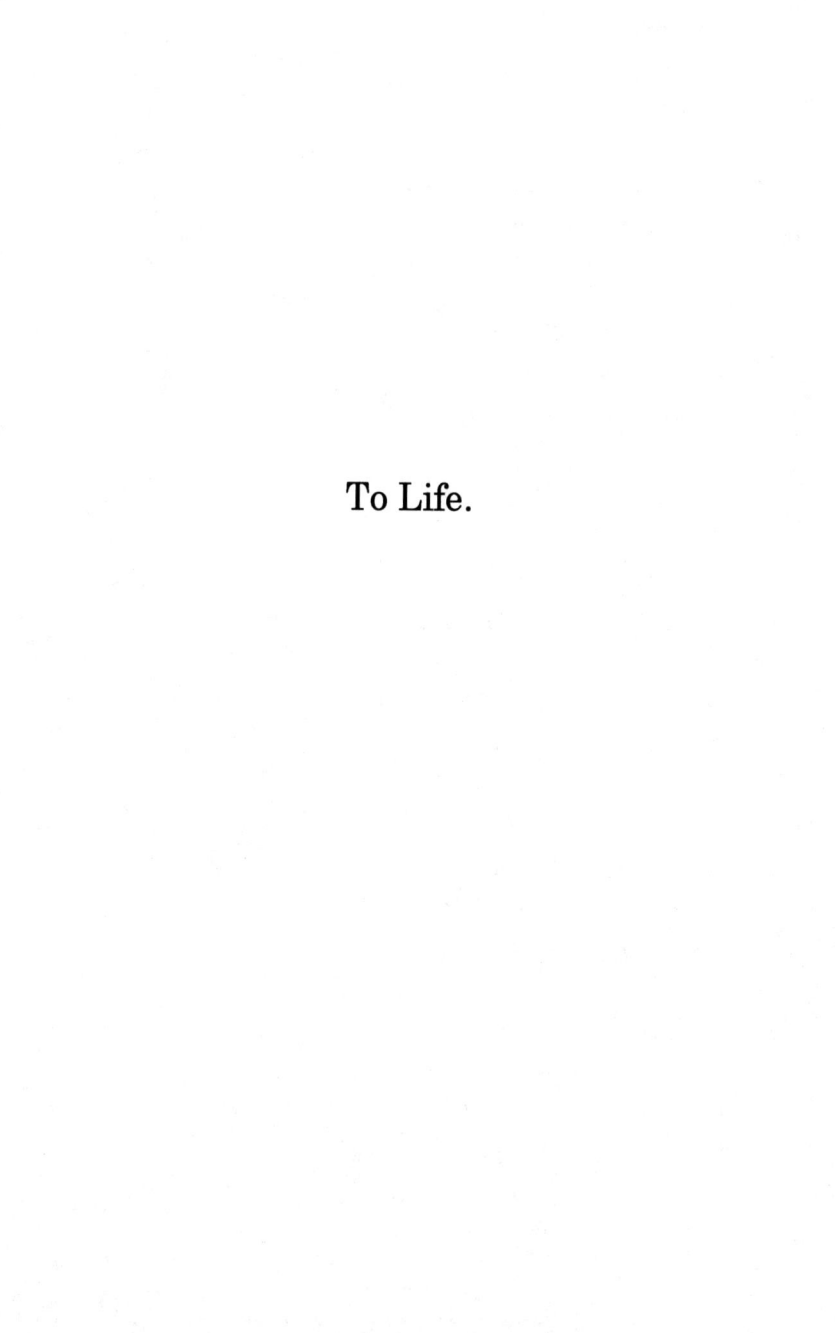

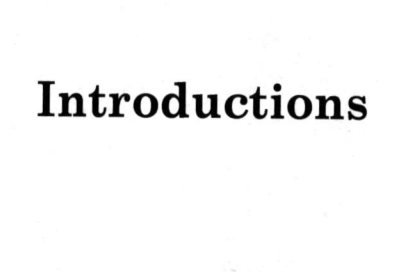

Introductions

Editor's Introduction

Those of you who read *Satan's Advice to Young Lawyers* know that I owe my success as an attorney to the advice I received from Satan. You also know that he has become my mentor and close confidant. I trust him implicitly.

So, when I learned that my wife was pregnant with our first child, I naturally asked Satan if he had any parenting advice. I only expected a few anecdotes and aphorisms. Instead, he told me: "This is a very important stage of your life. I will think on this question and provide you with a response when I am able."

As the weeks passed and my wife's belly grew larger, I wondered if he had forgotten or had found more important things to do. I should not have worried.

About two weeks before our child was born, Satan arrived at my law office, posing as a client, which was his typical disguise. He brought with him a small manuscript bound neatly in a red clasp folder.

"Here," he said, thrusting the folder towards me.

I reached out and took it. On the cover, written in thick black cursive, were the words: "Advice for the New Parent."

I put the folder down on my desk. "Thank you," I said.

He sat down in a leather chair, the cushions compressing under his weight. "When you asked me for parenting advice, I was not sure how I was going to respond. It was, believe it or not, a novel inquiry."

"I will read it tonight."

"Good," he said. "Be sure to share it with your wife. Parenting is much easier when it is a team effort."

I nodded.

"Have you thought of a name for your boy?"

I was momentarily surprised he knew it was going to be a boy, but then remembered who was sitting in the chair across from me. "No. I'd name him after you, but that might raise a few too many eyebrows."

He laughed. "I appreciate the sentiment, Aleister, but I believe you are correct."

"Maybe Henry or Joseph. We like traditional names."

He interlaced his fingers, resting his chin on them. He looked sad. "I too like them best. Put Gabriel in the mix, why don't you? I have always liked that name."

"Of course, I will mention it to my wife tonight."

"Good," he said, standing up quickly. "I must go now."

I stood too. "No time for a drink? I have some of that Scotch you like."

"I appreciate it," he said. "But, I fear I am called away on an urgent matter."

"I understand. Thank you for the advice," I said, gesturing at the folder on my desk.

He looked at me with kind eyes, a kindness I suppose few who meet him ever have the privilege of seeing. "You will be a good parent, Aleister. I do not plan on meeting your children in the afterlife."

A chill ran down my spine. "I hope you are right."

He smiled, opened the door and left the office.

That same evening, I read the advice. It was cogent and concise. There was no attempt at political correctness, only truth based on thousands of years of observation and practice. This was better than any of those four hundred-page baby advice tomes.

The next day, I gave it to my wife to read. I told her I found it in an antique shop. She was skeptical at first, but the certainty of the words won her over.

Our first child, Gabriel, is now two years old, and Satan's advice has served us well. Our boy may not always act like his namesake, but we can tell he is growing to be a confident boy who we hope will be a confident man.

My wife is pregnant again with a girl, due in three months as I write this. We have not chosen a name yet, but are leaning towards Mary. In anticipation of her birth, I went through my files looking for Satan's "Advice for the New Parent" so that I could re-read it.

It struck me that this advice should be shared with all parents. It makes the unknown road ahead much less frightening.

With Satan's blessing, I now offer you an unabridged version of his parenting advice.

No strings attached.

Aleister Lovecraft
San Francisco, February 2015

Satan's Introduction

When Aleister asked permission to publish my parenting advice, I granted it on the condition that I could write this brief introduction.

I recall feeling honored when Aleister asked me for parenting advice. After watching his career as an attorney blossom by following my advice in that area of his life, I knew that he would pay attention to what I have to say.

Aleister's request was, in fact, the first time anyone has ever thought to ask me for parenting advice. It strikes me as strange that there have been no prior requests, as who better than I to tell of lives gone awry and how those lives might have been saved?

I cannot, of course, blame every misguided life on bad parenting; there are simply too many variables in the world for such a simplistic explanation to be reliable. Nevertheless, I do blame a majority of wasted lives on parental missteps.

For those of you who may be skeptical, I want to make it clear that I do have the best interests of your children at heart. I do not want any more residents of my infernal prison. If there were no need for a keeper (and punisher) of lost souls, then I would be freed to return to my place in heaven with the rest of the angels, at the side of God.

I hope you will take this advice to heart and consider what I have to say very carefully. Your child's fate depends on it.

The One Thing

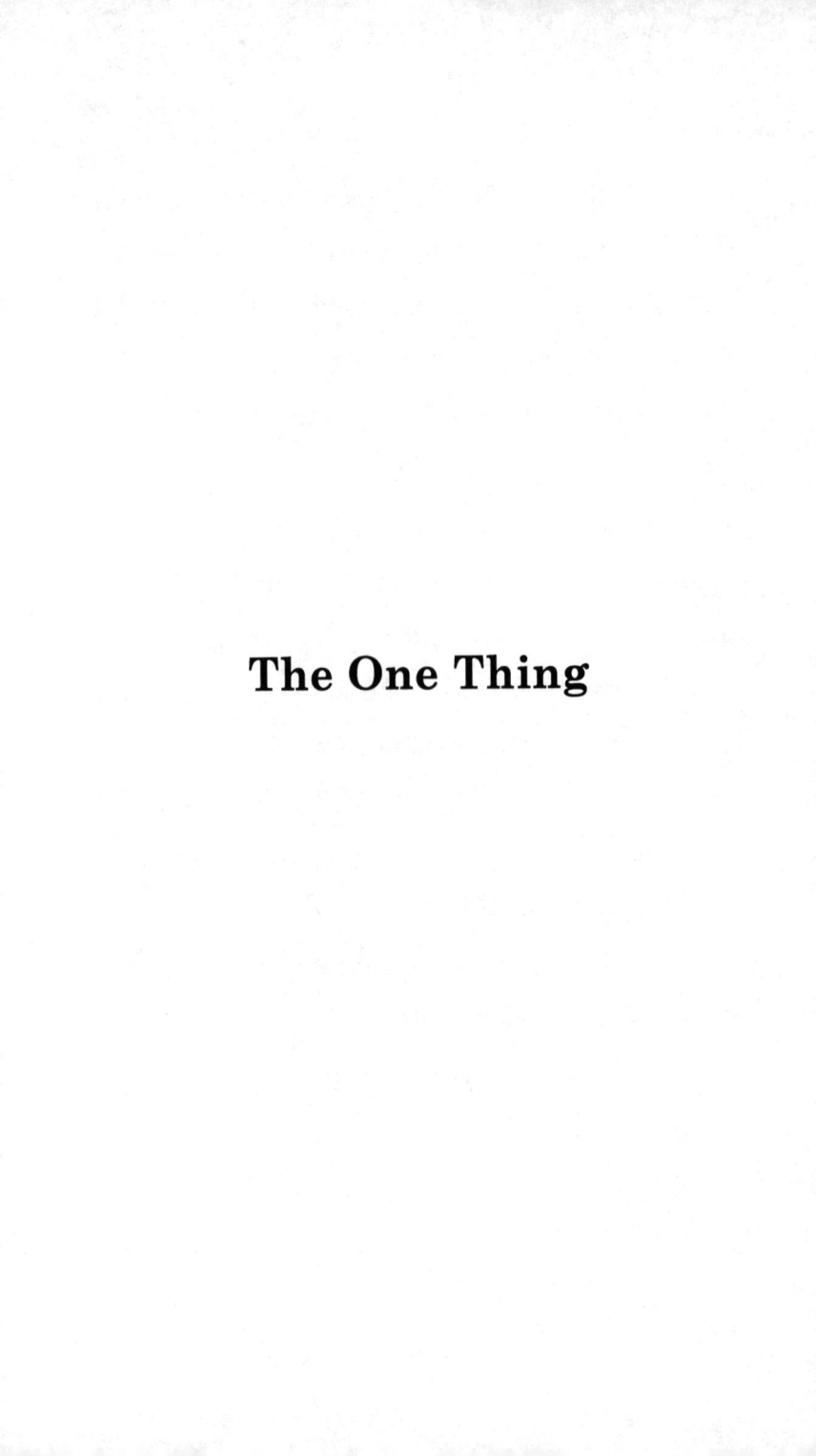

There is one simple thing you can do as a parent that will take care of ninety percent of parenting mistakes: Offer your child your unconditional love.

It sounds simple when I say it, but most people are simply incapable of *unconditional* love. That is why I have no shortage of guests in my abode.

In contrast, *conditional* love is just about the easiest thing a parent can offer a child. We love anything that makes us happy or satisfies some inner need. It is effortless to love a child when he is obedient or when she draws you a beautiful picture.

But, what about the child who screams at you, who disappoints you, who tells you in no uncertain terms that he hates you? It was your choice to create a life and bring it into the world. Your obligation to that life is unending allegiance and unconditional love. No. Matter. What.

Why?

Humans have a need for security. Without security, they develop all manner of neuroses and violent behaviors. They lash out at the world that seeks to hurt or destroy them. They suspect enemies where there are none. They become deformed in all possible ways and are incapable of reaching even ten percent of their potential.

Unconditional love gives your child a place of security. It allows your child to experience the world knowing that he can always return to you for support and regeneration. The world is a harsh place, filled with predators, violence and foolishness. Your child will get hurt – emotionally more often than physically – over and over again, but if he can come to you and receive love, he will survive the injury and recover even stronger.

This means that you will have to love your child in circumstances where the rest of the world finds your child to be unlovable.

When you become a parent, you understand what a truly difficult job God has. Is it really possible to love humanity when it does such awful things?

The true test of a parent is that moment when a little voice inside your head says, "Why did I have this child?" You can succumb to that voice, remain disappointed with your child, and let her know how much you despise her. Or, you can answer the question, "Because I love this child, and I must let her know that now and always."

You will have to answer this question many times as a parent. There will be times when your child rejects you outright, and still you must love your child.

Get this right, or else!

Part I: Pregnancy, Birth & Infancy

Pregnancy

Maternity is a matter of fact; Paternity is a matter of opinion. – Proverb.

I am an old-fashioned demi-god. I believe in traditional virtues and vices. I also believe that *women* get pregnant, *couples* do not.

So, please, if you are a man announcing the exciting news of your impending fatherhood to others, stop saying that ridiculous and offensive phrase, "*We* are pregnant." **No.** Your wife (or girlfriend[1]) is

---

[1] I realize that many societies no longer frown on out-of-wedlock births. I am not against them per se, but I am against people (mainly men) ignoring their duty to raise the children they have created. For many men, especially younger men, the yoke of marriage is what is needed to hold them to their duty. If, however, they can honor this duty without marriage, then, I suppose, marriage becomes superfluous.

pregnant. She is going to do all the hard work for the next nine months.

And, to the women reading this book, why would you ever submit to such pandering paternalistic propaganda and use a phrase like "we are pregnant"? Please, take some credit for growing a life inside of you. It is an extraordinary act that should not be dismissed by sharing credit with a sperm donor.

As to pregnancy itself, I have very limited advice, but it is important.

First, seek out the latest information in nutritional knowledge and eat the most healthy foods possible. Women should eat whatever is recommended for healthy fetal brain and body development.

It is of great concern to me that the nutritional value of foods available to many mothers is so poor. A century of industrial agriculture has led to a massive increase in available calories, but to a resultant decrease in the nutritional value of each calorie. I recommend eating organic fruits and vegetables and pastured or wild meats.

Second, complete any pending projects before the birth. Unless you have had a child before, you really have no idea how much time it takes to raise a child. If you have plans to take some classes, learn a new skill, write a book, etc., get it done *now*.

For those of you without children who think you have no free time now, you are completely, unequivocally, and irretrievably wrong. Stop watching TV, stop going out to bars, stop shopping all the time and get your task done.

Third, spend some time with your friends now, you won't be seeing much of them after the baby is born. Unless your friends have children, they will not understand your sudden unavailability after the birth. They may distance themselves from you. Not out of malice, but simply because you cannot be spontaneous any more. Prepare yourself for changing relationships.

Birth

You humans say birth is a miracle, but miracles are things that defy explanation. And, we all know where babies come from, don't we? Still, if you insist on calling it a miracle, then at least admit it is a messy and widely-available miracle.

I will not bother trying to explain what a typical birth is like. It is different for everyone. Some women can push a baby out in thirty minutes or less, while it takes hours or even days for other women. Just go where it takes you.

Beyond the physical process, each woman and man brings their unique emotions and life experience into the situation. Some people cry, others smile, some get startlingly angry and some simply pass out.

Birth is about bringing a new life into the world, sure, but what birth really does is reveal who you are as a human being. Until the creation of birth control a few decades ago, birth was a nearly universal experience for women who lived to adulthood. Similarly, fatherhood was a nearly universal experience for men. The ability of birth control to prevent pregnancy so effectively has severed you humans from your own humanity.

Birth is a liminal experience *par excellance*: Once you go through it, you are never the same.

Participation in the birth process is part of becoming a complete human being. People who do not have children are incomplete human beings. Sure, they walk upright and have an exceptionally large cerebral cortex, but that is not what makes one human. A human is only human by virtue of his or her understanding of those who have lived before.

Childless humans have no idea of the emotions birth[2] and parenting stir within the soul. These empty husks of humanity will often judge you as a parent without any idea how difficult it is. *After all*, they think smugly, *my fluffy little dog is well-behaved, why can't those people control that child?* Rest assured, such people are laying the pavers of their personal road to perdition.

After your baby is born and you hold the new life in your hands, all of the possibilities and dangers of the world suddenly manifest themselves within your mind. You hope (and maybe pray) that your child will reach her full

---

[2] I do not doubt that adoptive parents can love their children unconditionally. However, there is something *sui generis* about going through the birth process that I believe simply cannot be replicated.

potential and change the world, and you fear (and maybe curse) the countless dangers lurking everywhere, from childhood accidents to terrorist attacks to epidemics.

Do not dwell on these fears as your child is born. Let the current of emotion wash over you. Do not let worry spoil this – or any other – moment for you. This moment that you will remember for the rest of your life, whether empires fall or you one day travel to distant and mysterious lands, the memory of your child's birth will never fade.

Having become a parent, the deepest wisdom of humanity is now available for your understanding. You need only look and want to see it.

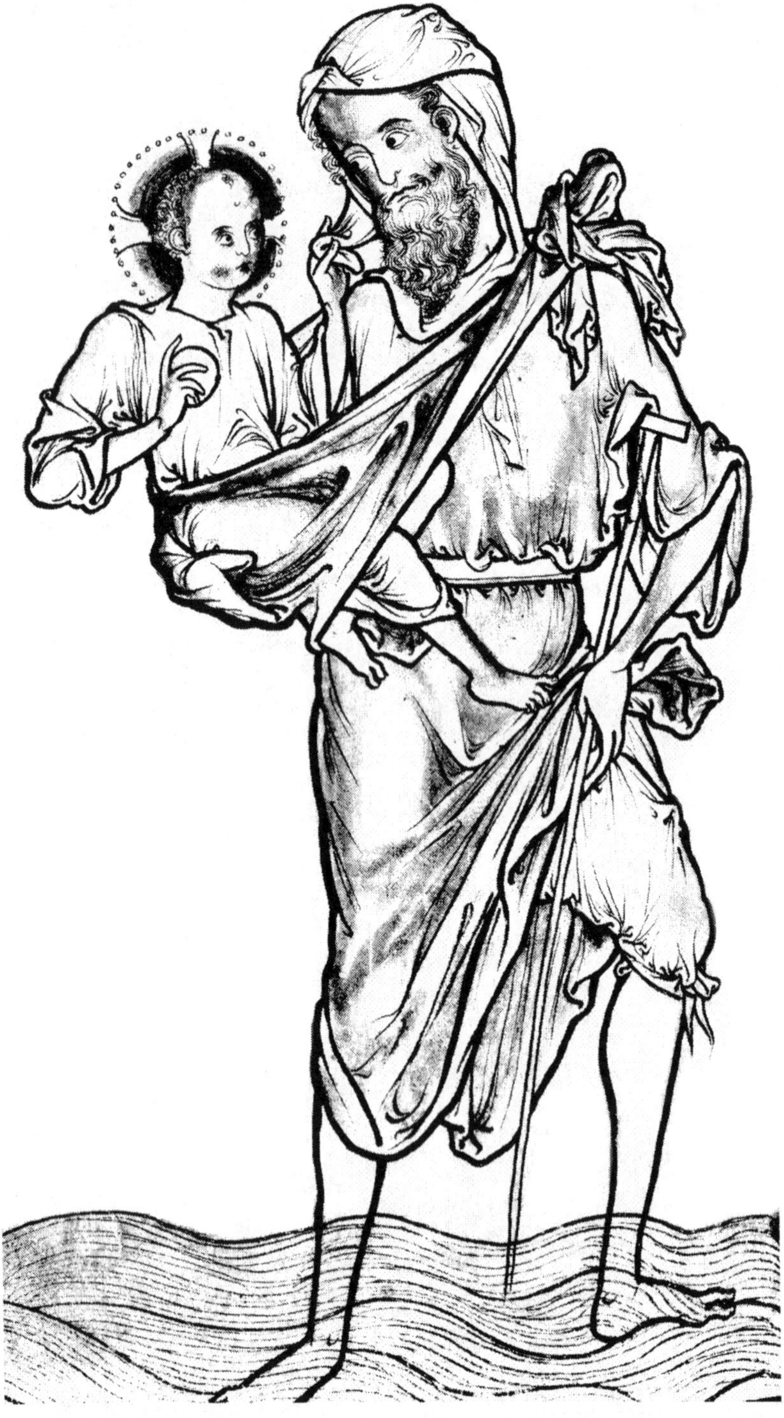

How to Deal with Your Newborn

"There are one hundred and fifty-two distinctly different ways of holding a baby – and all are right." – Heywood Broun.

I have spent countless hours observing babies during my lifetime, usually when misguided parents perform an occult ceremony to summon me to ask that I make their baby into my disciple. These fools fail to realize I only make contracts with souls that have reached the age of majority. But, since they have called me to their home in the correct manner, I often stay a while, watching the forlorn and damned parents in their futile contortions of summoning, a preview of their afterlife.

I also watch the baby.

During the first months after its birth, the baby does little that is recognizably human. This can be maddening – literally – for some parents. The baby does not smile or laugh, it just stares with its big, bulgy alien eyes seated within its tiny, spongy head.

Eventually, the baby gains greater control of its neck muscles and its brain starts working better, and something else happens: it starts looking around. A lot. Like a tweaker on meth.

The baby is learning, similar to the manner in which a highly-evolved extraterrestrial who lands on earth can take everything in and begin speaking the language of the country in which it lands within minutes. Sadly, human babies are not so highly-evolved and take years to develop speech. Still, what you say and do with, to, and in front of the baby at this time matters greatly.

I am not a developmental pediatrician, but thousands of years of observations have taught me a few things about raising babies.

First, when you speak with your baby, you must use proper grammar and diction. No baby talk. Peek-a-boo and silly games like that are fine, but when you speak to the baby, speak properly. It follows that you should read books to your baby with complete sentences. These books need not be complicated. I am thinking of *Goodnight Moon*, for instance. But, feel free to read something more exciting, like *The Odyssey* or *Blood Meridian*.

Second, play with the baby as often as possible. This is hard work for some modern parents who would prefer to stare at an electronic device rather than interact with a human being. If you are one of those pathetic people, get over it or get into treatment. Remember, idle hands are the devil's plaything, and if you teach your baby that you do not have time for him now, then when he is a teenager, I will be seeing a lot of him.

Please understand, I do realize some humans have limits on how long they can be around a baby; it can get boring and monotonous. When you need a break, enlist the help of grandparents or friends to give you a few hours' respite.

Third, keep all wireless electronics away from your infant. These devices give off *radiation*. Do not let your baby play with your cell phone, preferably at all, but only in airplane mode as a backup plan.

Fourth, get your child outside as often as possible. It does not matter if this is your own backyard, a park, the beach, the desert, the mountains, or whatever. Let your baby get dirty, stare at bugs, and roll around on the dirt. Not only will your child benefit from getting outside, but so will you. I have watched humans for millennia, and I have noticed a sadness descend upon many of you who do not get outside and look at trees and animals and bushes. You have gone away from your origins in nature and have separated yourselves from the place you came from. I see your collective mental health suffering for it. Without enough exposure to the natural world, humanity's future is bleak.

That is really it.

For those of you with short attention spans, I can boil all this down to a single sentence: Spend as much quality time as possible with your newborn in order to give your child the best foundation for a happy and successful life.

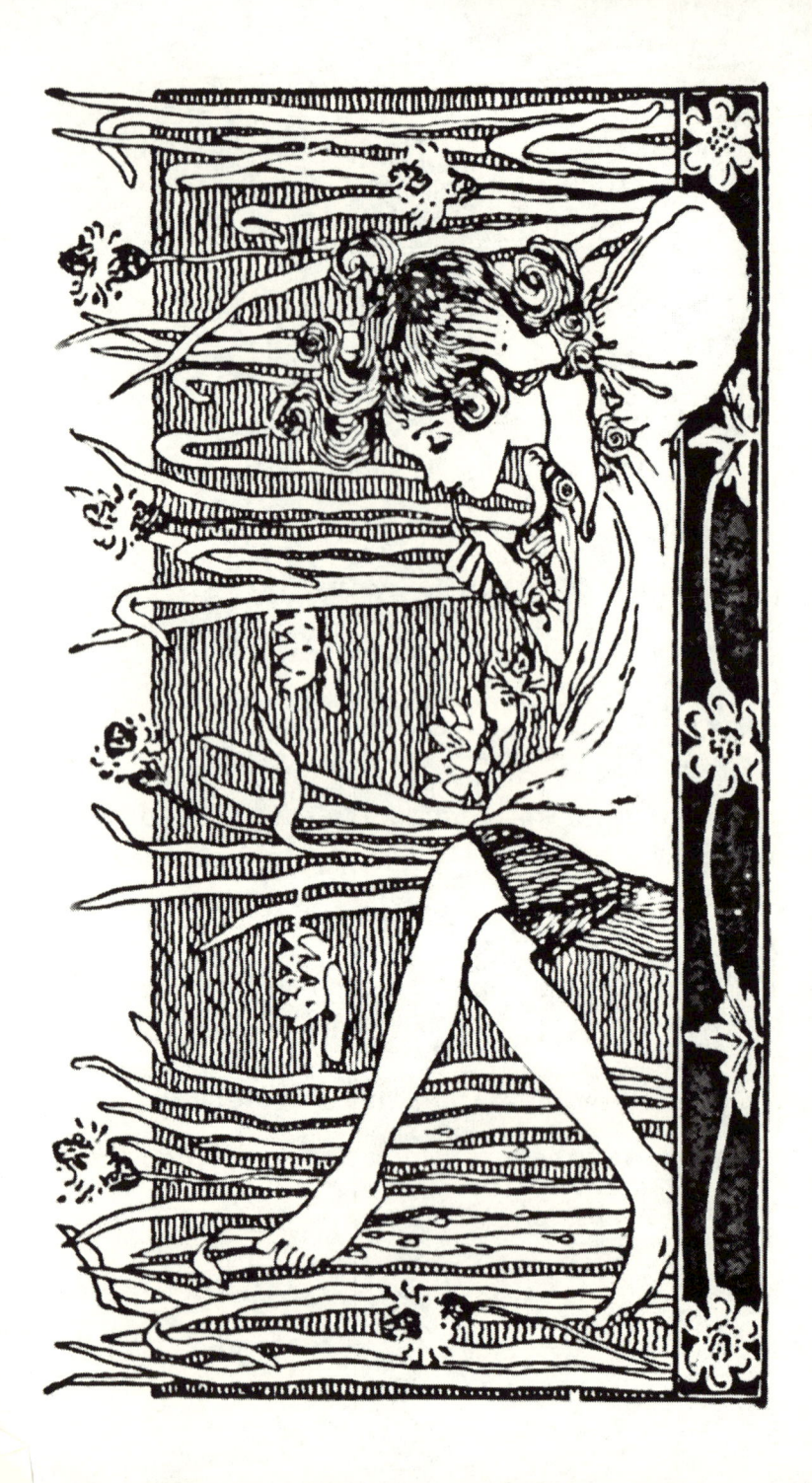

Sleeping

"There was never a child so lovely but his mother was glad to get him asleep." – Ralph Waldo Emerson.

Parents, especially first-time parents, obsess over the sleep habits of their newborns. People who have older children will ask you, "Is your baby sleeping through the night yet?"

The sleep of an infant is a revelation for new parents. It is so quiet. Most new parents will check their baby's breathing multiple times per night for the first few weeks to reassure themselves that the baby is still alive. The breathing is nearly imperceptible at times.

The questions and anxieties about sleep go beyond breath, of course. Some common questions are: Should I put my baby on his back or stomach when I put him down to sleep? Should I swaddle my baby? Should the baby's room be hot or cold for optimal sleep? How close to bedtime should the final feeding be?

I have no idea about the answers to those questions. Consult a doctor or a book about what to expect from your infant. All I know is that I have seen parents around the world answer these questions in every conceivable way, and their children usually make it to adulthood. There indeed may be an ideal answer to all of these questions, but I would not worry about it too much.

Instead of answering these questions, I will tell you instead the three most common mistakes I see leading to long-term sleep problems for children. Ignore these at your peril.

The first mistake I see is parents sleeping with their babies for too long after their birth. I see nothing wrong with having your baby sleep in a crib in the same room with you or in your bed with you for the first few weeks of its life. It is calming for the baby and reassures the new parents that the baby is safe. And, it is very common throughout history to use such an arrangement.

Nevertheless, at a minimum, get the baby out of your bed within four weeks of birth. Failure to do this leads to horrible attachment issues for the child and sleep disturbances in the years to come. Ideally at this time, you will move the baby to her own room or, at least, as far away from your bed as possible in your bedroom. At the end of eight weeks, the baby should be in her own room, unless you live in a small apartment.

The second mistake I see is when parents rush into the baby's room within an instant of hearing it cry. Such responsiveness is common and expected during the first few weeks of life, but after that, the baby should learn to take care of itself.

I advocate the "cry it out" regime. It may seem heartless to let a baby cry for ten or fifteen minutes, but unless the baby is sick, there is really no need to come to his aid. You cannot give in. It only makes it worse if you resist for ten minutes and then go to the baby. Should you do this, you succeed only in training the baby that it will take ten minutes of crying to summon you. Either be a patsy and rush in immediately, or stand your ground no matter the cost.

The third mistake I see is not putting the baby to sleep until you are ready to go to sleep yourself. This creates huge problems as your baby grows older because you do not get any time to yourself in the evening. Your child will begin to feel entitled to stay up as late as you, and eventually, you will have great difficulty ordering the child to go to bed. A battle of wills at the end of the day is never enjoyable.

To avoid this dark future, put your baby on a sleep schedule as soon as your baby is sleeping through the night. Put her to sleep at the same time each night, preferably one or two hours before you want to sleep. That way, you have some personal time to read, to watch TV, or maybe even to get busy making your next baby.

Feeding

"Feeding a baby is like filling a hole with putty – you get it in and then you sort of shave off all the excess around the hole and get it back in, like you're spackling." –
Anne Lamott.

Let us face facts, a new baby is just a food tube. It needs enough nutrients to grow and keep its brain functioning properly. If it is hungry, it will let you know by crying and screaming until it passes out or you feed it.

The simplest mechanism for satiating your precious food tube is breast-feeding. I will not provide you with any advice about how to get the baby to "latch" on, what to do about painful, engorged breasts, or which mechanical pump works best for storing breast milk. You are on your own there.

I will warn nursing women to beware that whatever you eat, your baby will eat a few hours later in the form of your breast milk. So, if you eat a gigantic bean and cheese burrito with lots of hot salsa, do not be surprised if your baby gets very gassy a few hours later. If you eat a lot of greens at one meal, do not be surprised if your baby's poop becomes watery and green. It is like a parlor trick.

I will also refrain from any recommendations about baby formula. Do your research and get one that your baby keeps down. I have heard that certain plant-based formulas are not favored, but I really do not keep up on the science of nutrition. Important here: Do not believe anything a manufacturer of formula tells you; get your information from a third-party source.

The feeding of a young baby is really quite boring. For me, the most amusing part of childhood is watching parents start giving solid food to their babies.

The angst in selecting jars of baby food is palpable. Parents read labels, ponder, and fuss. Will my child like pureed peas or potatoes? The bananas or the fruit medley?

Recall, will you, that jarred baby food did not exist until the last 100 years. So, how did babies eat before then? Did they breastfeed until they had all their teeth? The answer is no. (Well, among some people, that sort of thing *is* fashionable.) So, what did they eat?

In the old days, people would just take whatever it was they were eating, mash it up or pass it through a food mill, and then feed it to the child. No expensive little jars of flavorless mashed goo, but a tasty mix of whatever was on the table.

Is it any wonder that so many children reject the nasty vegetables in baby food jars?

Most of these vegetables have been boiled and mashed, with no salt or any spices of any kind added. Try a spoonful of this crap for yourself sometime. I would not feed it to my hell hounds.

Why are so many parents afraid to feed their children actual, real *food*? Why do they turn to packaged dreck? I have no idea. Please, just stop it. You are giving your child all the wrong signals.

Feeding your child something different from what you are eating subtly tells the child that he is different. Maybe he will take this to mean he is special, or maybe he will take this to mean he is unwanted. Neither of these is a good outcome.

Think of the children who have been breastfed. Each meal they had from birth until solid foods are introduced had nuance and flavor depending on what their mother had eaten earlier. How confusing it must be for such a child to go from a rainbow of flavors to the eternal flavorlessness of prison slop. They must be asking, "Is the world of adults all so boring and monotonous?" (I note here that formula-fed children have been used to monotony in their food from birth, so the change will not be as much a shock for them. But, is that a good thing?)

One thing you will notice, if you feed your child jarred food, is that she loves the fruit and hates the vegetables. The reason should be obvious: sugar. Fruit has a lot of sugar in it, and just because it is "natural" does not mean it is good. Soon enough, your child will learn to refuse the vegetables and gobble the fruit. You, as a tired parent, will give in and purchase more and more fruit flavors. Your child will grow to love sugar, and the end result will be a child conditioned to need sugar

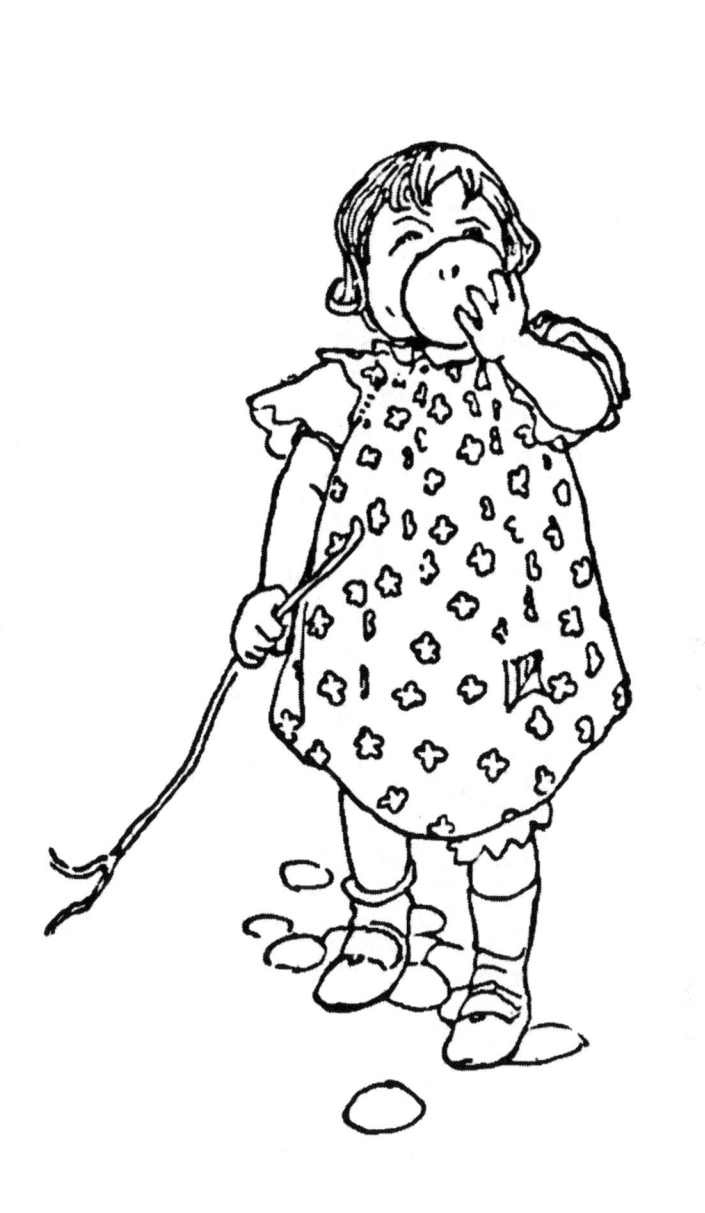

with every meal. This is why feeding your child mashed versions of what you eat is better because she will learn that dinner time is surprising and will look forward to eating tasty things.

The introduction of solid food to your child's diet is one of life's great amusements. You will notice that, as your child begins learning how to eat, more of the food finds a home on his face or bib than in his mouth. It is natural, and your child is not to be scolded. The coordination of the chewing and swallowing reflex is not an easy one, especially for a food tube who has been doing nothing but sucking and swallowing for its entire life.

Be patient. Take pictures. Laugh a lot.

Mealtime should bring out camaraderie and conversation. It is a playful and wonderful time for humans. Teach your child this by example.

Diapers

"Diaper backward spells repaid. Think about it." – Marshall McLuhan.

Be grateful that you live in modern times.

As a result of my immortality, I take the long view on humanity. Believe me, when it comes to diapers, you have it easy.

Back in the old days, you would be lucky to have even cloth diapers. More than likely you would have had to use leaves, animal skin, moss, or even nothing. Imagine your little "bundle of joy" peeing and pooping at will. Imagine the clean up. Imagine the slipping hazard.

The number one rule, when it comes to changing diapers is: do your part.

I see lots of couples get into battles when it comes to changing diapers. Yes, it can be gross, but mainly it is just a brief interruption to your day. Take turns between parents. If you never help change diapers, then you are not much of a parent. (This does not apply to you if you are rich and have a full-time nanny. And, in any event, if you have a nanny, why are you bothering to read this book? The nanny is the real parent, not you.)

When you have your first baby, I know most of you will be clueless about how to change a diaper. It might take you a few minutes. It might frustrate you, especially when you have to do it in the middle of the night. Just take a deep breath (or maybe not so deep, depending on the gift you unwrap) and get through it.

Make fair compromises with your spouse on changing diapers. If one parent is the breadwinner and needs to wake up early, then the non-breadwinning parent should change the diapers at night during the workweek. The breadwinning parent can change the majority of diapers on the weekend.

This next paragraph is mainly for the male readers. Men, it is you – in the majority of couples I have observed – who try to avoid diaper changing duty. Most of you justify this by deeming baby-related chores as "women's work." If that is what you truly think, then you need to live your entire married life in the role of the dominant patriarch, enduring all stress for your family and giving your wife gifts while you impose rules and structure. If, as is more likely, you are just being a lazy, pain-in-the-ass who purports to believe that women should be the equals of men, then live up to your sloganeering and change some damn diapers.

Finally, please do not discuss your diaper-changing adventures with non-parents. They will not understand why you are so interested in the shape, size, or smell of your child's bowel movements.[3] They do not want to hear about how little Johnny looked like he had a duck's tail because his diaper was so full of urine. Keep that stuff to yourself.

---

[3] But, if a poo smear resembles Jesus, be sure to call the news outlets, as they love running stories about things like that. (Confidentially, just between you and me, the extant depictions of Jesus look nothing like the man.)

Illness

Most parents dread the first time – and then every subsequent time – their baby gets sick. There is good reason for this: sick babies are horrid. I was going to say evil, but that would be unfair. Evil implies choice.

A sick baby cannot tell you he is sick other than by screaming and crying at the top of his lungs. To ensure that you heard him, he will not sleep at all during the night, but will fall asleep just as the sun comes up. The baby does this so that he will be well rested in order to scream and cry all the next night.

In addition to being horrid, sick babies are sloppy. It is bad enough that a healthy baby cannot control its urination and defecation, but a sick baby adds green snot and (sometimes) streams of vomit to those foul things. Every parent has a story of checking on their screaming baby in the middle of the night and finding the baby covered in diarrhea, vomit and snot. You will not escape.

A sick baby will not give you a break. If you pick her up to comfort her and she quiets, she will begin screaming again the moment you set her down. It is okay to ignore the baby for a few minutes in order to have a moment to yourself to sip coffee (or whiskey). The baby is trying to manipulate you to do her will. The manipulation is not out of malice, but merely out of the self-preservation instinct with which all humans are born.

When you have a sick baby, you are forced to adjust yourself to the oscillations of the screaming and crying. When there is screaming and crying, you comfort the baby as best you can. When there is not, you take a nap. Do not try to accomplish any goals other than keeping yourself and your baby alive. If the illness lasts more than twenty-four hours, you will be in a catatonic-like state where all pretense of higher thought has been stripped away.

With a sick baby, you must take things as they come, put one foot in front of the other, and live.

Discipline of Infants

"Children are completely egotistic; they feel their needs intensely and strive ruthlessly to satisfy them." – Sigmund Freud.

Infants should not be disciplined – ever. Discipline is a form of behavior control, necessary only for those who understand good and evil, right and wrong. Infants are without guile, and therefore the justification for their discipline does not exist.

I have watched countless hapless parents yell at, spank and even beat infants. The ignorant and despicable acts of these clueless people reveals starkly their self-loathing and their misunderstanding of infants. Let me enlighten you now so that you do not make these same abominable mistakes, which may irreparably damage your child and will – with certainty – open the gates of hell for you in the afterlife.

The purpose of human infancy is to explore the world, mainly for the purpose of understanding human society and the laws of physics.

An infant is interested in everything it sees. It watches how adults walk, talk and interact. It wants to grab, pull and taste everything. I once told Gabriel, before I was sent away from heaven, that it seemed as if infants do everything in their power to kill themselves as their exasperated parents rush around trying to prevent disaster. He laughed. I miss Gabriel's laugh.

And so, your child is simply exploring the world, like a puppy exploring a new yard. Your job is to supervise, not to discipline. If your child gets into danger, do not scold the child, but warn the child to be careful or to avoid putting its fingers in the electric socket. Think of the mother cat who grabs her kittens by the neck to reposition them when they get too far away from her. She does not cuff them; instead, she makes it easier for her to supervise their activities. If you start to feel anger toward your baby for its explorations, let the mother cat be your example.

If you discipline your child for its curiosity or out of rage that you cannot watch television uninterrupted, you are instilling fear and uncertainty in your child. This is simply the worst thing you can do. It increases the odds your child will grow up with some form of neurosis and live a life of undeserved mediocrity.

Such senseless discipline begins the process of destroying your child's natural inborn growth mindset and replacing it with a fixed mindset, which predisposes your child for failure and lifelong disappointment. If you have not heard about these types of mindsets[4], let me enlighten you.

With a fixed mindset, one believes one's basic qualities, like talent, intelligence or ability in a particular area, are simply fixed traits. Such people spend their time documenting their talent or intelligence instead of developing them. They wrongly believe talent is the *sine qua non* of success and that success should, therefore, be effortless. Anytime people with a fixed

---

[4] These two categories of mindset were popularized by a Stanford psychologist named Carol Dweck. Though, we demi-gods have observed them for millennia, we never bothered to reveal them to you. (As a side note, I find the term "mindset" utterly offensive. It implies stagnation and a lack of plasticity. It undermines the very free will given to humans by their creator. It turns humans into automatons. But, I suppose we are stuck with that term, for now, as a shorthand.)

mindset are unable to perform a task on the first attempt, they immediately think they are stupid and give up. Do you want your child to be a quitter who hates himself?

Someone with a growth mindset believes his or her most basic abilities can be developed through hard work, dedication and perseverance. Intelligence and talent help, but work is what makes all the difference. People with a growth mindset tend to have much greater resilience and can endure more trying times and hardship to reach their goals. Sounds good, right?

And so, you should allow your infant to do whatever he or she feels like, so long as it does not pose a danger to that child's life and limb, or to the life and limb of others.

One of the more difficult parts of parenting is determining when the period of amoral infancy ends and when the manipulative toddler years begin. At that point, discipline is both justified and necessary.

Adults without Children

> *"All men know their children mean more than life. If childless people sneer – well, they've less sorrow. But what lonesome luck!"* – Euripides.

You will quickly learn that adults without children do not want to hear much about your baby. They view it as sad and pathetic that you seem incapable of speaking about anything other than your newborn child. It is incomprehensible to them that your child could possibly be so interesting. (What they fail to understand is that you are so sleep-deprived that you have no time or energy to watch the news, read a book, or keep up on the latest celebrity gossip.)

The bitter truth is, of course, that your child is no different from the billions of children who have been born during the millennia humans have roamed the earth. All babies cry, pee, poop, spit up, crawl and look cute.

Your child is not special, not when viewed from a distance. That is what the childless adult is thinking as you prattle on about how funny it was when your cute-as-a-button baby boy peed on your face while you were changing his diaper or when your widdle-snookems baby girl kept pulling on your ear while she was breastfeeding.

This is cringe worthy stuff for non-parents.

But, to you, your child means the world. People who have children understand; people who do not have children do not and cannot understand. Do not try and make them.

If other adults seem bored by talk of your child, then stop talking. If you have nothing else to say, then maybe you cannot be around other adults for a while. It is a sad truth that children end friendships, especially shallow friendships where the only thing you had in common was talking sports, going shopping, or getting drunk.

Parenthood can be an isolating experience. I have seen many parents, especially women who are stay-at-home mothers, become socially isolated and very sad. This was not true as much in the past, when family members would come and stay with the new parents to help them make the transition. Now, people often work until the baby is about to pop out, give birth, and then have no one around to help them. When their friends abandon them too, it can become overwhelming.

Do not give in to despair in such situations. Reach out to family to talk about your new baby. Get people to spend time with the baby so you can get out of the house and be an independent adult for a few hours. If you do not have these resources, then find a blog or two on the internet about being a new parent. Many of these are targeted towards women, but there is an increasing community of stay-at-home dads who have support on the internet too.

Just because the circle of friends that existed before the birth is shrinking does not mean you have to become a shut-in whose only purpose in life is to do the bidding of the little Id Monster you recently brought into the world.

Taking Time Off Work

If you are like most parents in the modern world, you work at a job that takes you away from your home for long periods of time. And, it is almost a certainty that your employer does not want you to bring a screaming baby to work with you.

In the old days, many new parents were farmers or self-employed artisans who could keep their children near them as they worked. After all, in the pre-modern age and in many places even today, new parents do not have the luxury of stopping work for weeks at a time to "bond" with their newborn.

In my observations, this older form of society was better for everyone, including newborns. Normally, female relatives would arrive for the birth and help the new mother through it. After the birth, some of these relatives would stay to help with the baby for a few days or weeks until the new mother was back to full strength. All the while, stories were shared about raising babies and clueless husbands. The newborn received quality care, the mother learned the generational wisdom, and the father was kept at a distance so as not to screw anything up.

In most "enlightened" modern societies, laws permit new parents to take some time off from work in order to bond with their baby and get used to being parents. These laws allow both men and women to take time off.

For women, the need for time is obvious. They need to recover physically, which for some will take a few days and others a few weeks. They also need to recover psychologically. Many women go temporarily insane after having a baby. The baby has sucked most of their brain tissue out of their bodies in order to form its own brain, so the architecture of the woman's brain is damaged. Furthermore, the woman's hormones are oscillating wildly and creating mood swings of geological proportions. No one wants a person like this at work.

But, the troubling part about the weeks and months a woman may take off from work is her feeling of isolation. If no relatives or friends visit during those early weeks, she is often alone with the strange, expressionless creature known as a newborn. It screams and cries and poops and pees and does not smile. It can be disheartening. I have seen some new mothers driven to do horrible things by this isolation.

So, if you are a new mother planning to take time off, be sure that relatives and friends can visit with you. If they are not nearby, find a new mother's group to meet with once or twice per week. It really does take a village, or at least a small team, to raise a child. Modern society often forgets this.

For men, the need for time off is less obvious and is often discouraged. Men are not supposed to care much about newborn babies. Men cannot breast feed and tend to be more impatient than women. So, this line of thinking goes, what good are they around babies and why should they take time off work? I do not deny that many men are clueless around babies, and in fact, look for ways to remain that way in order to avoid some of the more tedious care of a newborn.

Nevertheless, it is a truism that men should be a presence in the lives of their children from the beginning. Even if they cannot feed a baby with their breasts, they should be present to assist the mother.

Babies notice these things: people helping others or being nice to others or ignoring others or harming others. You want your baby to know that you are a good person because you care about the one person in the world the baby loves without question: its mother.

When asking to take time off from work to "bond" with their new baby, men will have to deal with some lack of consideration, especially from older male bosses. If you are in this situation, do your best to ignore any snide comments, and enjoy your time off. If your boss mistreats you upon your return to work, you may want to mention to him that your baby bonding leave is protected by law and any retaliation for exercising that right is illegal. This will, I am certain, piss off your boss, but you need to stop this sort of behavior immediately. Besides, it makes great practice for disciplining your children as they grow.

Divorce Warning

"Infancy conforms to nobody; all conform to it." – Ralph Waldo Emerson.

Infancy is the time when many new parents get divorced.

I have seen it a lot in recent decades, as divorce became increasingly acceptable through the course of the twentieth century. Before then, new parents had no choice but to get through these tough times; divorce was simply not done. This is not to say that divorce is not needed for certain couples, especially where one or both partners are abusive and toxic.

Unfortunately, divorce during the infancy of children usually occurs for the wrong reasons. I am not opposed to divorce where the marriage is dysfunctional, but I am a traditionalist. In my opinion, marriage is a sacred bond, and it should be broken only when absolutely necessary. Indeed, it is the struggle through the difficult times that enables humans to grow and become wise.

In a typical infancy-divorce scenario, the new baby suddenly gets all of the attention. The parents do not get enough sleep. Tempers fray and putative realizations about each spouse occur to the other.

If you feel yourself heading in the direction of divorce, evaluate your feelings against the backdrop of this momentous shift in your life. Do you really want to get a divorce, or are you just reluctant to confront your new status as a parent and all the responsibility and sacrifice that comes with it?

Some of the common causes of divorce during a child's infancy are: battles over who will change the diapers, the breadwinner starts staying later at work to avoid parental responsibilities, one parent refuses to stop spending excessive amounts of money on frivolous personal items of no benefit to the family, one parent does not help with the baby at night, etc. These are mainly problems of maturity, not the basis for divorce.

Before you make the decision to get a divorce, ask a trusted friend or relative who is married and has children with his or her current spouse for an opinion about your situation. Describe what you think is the problem, and see what they have to say.

Part II: Toddlers

Toddlers

A toddler is a person who toddles or "moves with short unsteady steps while learning to walk or being excessively drunk."

I hope your young child is not drinking alcohol, so I think the first part of the definition applies. To me, a toddler can be anywhere from 12 months to 36 months. By the age of three, most children walk and run quite competently. At that point, you can just call them a child or a "little girl" or "little boy."

Discipline of Toddlers

"The rod and reproof give wisdom, but a child left to himself brings shame to his mother." – Proverbs 29:15

Unlike infants, toddlers require discipline. During this period of life, the child is developing its independence and its selfishness. This is when you hear "mine" and "no" for the first time, and the child really means it.

Exactly how to impose the discipline will vary with each child. I cannot give one-size-fits-all advice here, but I can tell you that most of the souls that dwell with me in the afterlife have had a violent or severely dysfunctional upbringing. I can say that violent discipline of a toddler is only effective in the short-term because it instills fear. In the long-term, such discipline creates severe and often intractable problems for the preteen, teenager and adult the child becomes.

Notwithstanding the hallowed quote at the start of this chapter, I do not condone the use of violence against children; it is wrong.

The conundrum for the parent is that most toddlers do not understand reason. They still live in the moment, like an infant; though, unlike an infant, they have developed a sense of self and the ability to express their irrational thoughts using language or force. If a toddler wants something, the toddler will take it without compunction. A long-winded explanation about sharing has no effect.

This also begs the question of whether you want to teach your child how to share at such a young age. Is teaching a toddler to "share" really not just teaching her how to be weak?

How to give away what she has acquired by her own wit or strength? Perhaps now is the time to instill the virtues of power and dominance. As the child matures and enters into the age of reason – around age five or six, you can begin to instill the virtues of charity and society.

I am not saying that you should allow your child to be a bully and to take what other children have without offering something in exchange. If you catch your child stealing something from another child or shoving another child to get what your child wants, you must step in and discipline your child. If you do not, you are teaching your child to use violence to get what he or she wants. This is unacceptable, just as using violence to discipline your child is unacceptable.

Instead, I am suggesting that the toddler stage is when you praise your child for his ability to acquire and master.

Confidence in one's ability to survive is a helpful trait for long-term success and for ensuring your child's inborn growth mindset is never crushed. If your child rushes in to daycare and grabs her favorite toy before anyone else can, praise her. If your child grabs all the hidden Easter eggs before the other kids do, praise your child's skill and speed, don't make him share the bounty of his abilities with the others.

The "Playdate"

If there is one word I hate more than any in the modern parenting lexicon, it is "playdate."

Whatever happened to "going to Bill's house" or "going to play with Becky" or something like that? Everything is arranged and structured. Children cannot even have fun anymore unless it comports to the schedules of their parents, who must also be present for the "playdate."

Just read the explanation of "playdate" from Wikipedia and tell me it doesn't make you want to puke in your mouth:

> **Play date** or **playdate** is an expression primarily used in the US for an arranged appointment for

children to get together for a few hours to play. Play dates have become common because the work schedules for busy parents, along with media warnings about leaving children unattended, prevent the kind of play that children of other generations participated in. Play dates are also arranged by destinations that feature child-friendly programs like museums, parks or playgrounds. The intention of a play date is to give children time to interact freely in a less structured environment than other planned activities might provide. Play dates are different from organized activities or scheduled sports, because they are not usually structured. Play dates are becoming part of the vernacular of popular culture and form a part of children's "down time". Most parents prefer children to use these hours to form friendships by playing with other children either one-on-one or within small groups. When children are very young, most parents stay for the play date and use the time to form their own friendships and parental alliances.

Parental alliances? Down time? Not *usually* structured? Demonic.

I understand that parents are afraid of the freaks that lurk in the world. Believe me, I know they are there because they all end up with me in the afterlife. But, please, do not live your life in fear and do not instill a fear of freedom and random acts of playtime in your children.

The possibilities of childhood and the childish imagination are vast and amazing, but these possibilities are stifled and smothered by the imposition of brief windows of time for such activities, making them just another checkbox on the to-do list of a mundane life.

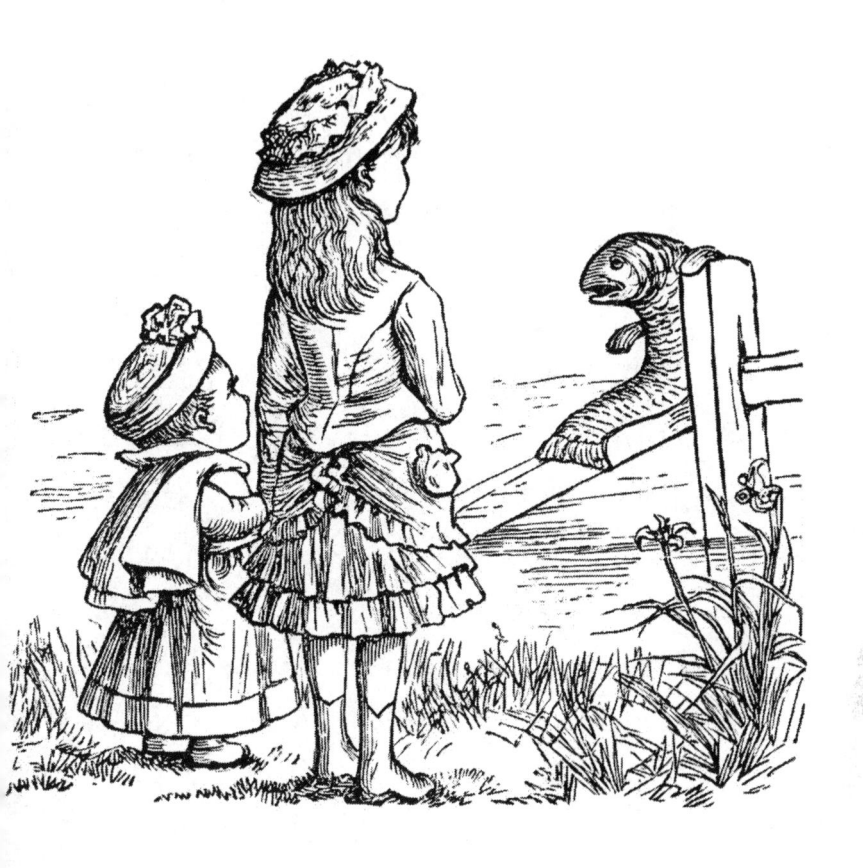

Toilet Training

This is as confusing a time for children as it is for parents. I address this topic as a FAQ, rather than in narrative fashion to reduce the confusion to a minimum.

Q: When is my child ready for toilet training?
A: The first thing to understand about toilet (or potty) training is not to rush it. Normally, you should start when your child is old enough to understand what you are telling it *and* your child quickly becomes uncomfortable having a steaming pile of smelly crap in its diaper. That is the main difference between a child who is ready for toilet training versus one who is not.

Q: How long will it take?

A: It varies. Some children get it right away and are diaper-free within a few weeks. Other children may take months to understand the signals from their body and get to a toilet on time. When it takes a child a long time to learn, it could be for a variety of reasons, including not being ready, mixed signals from parents and caretakers, fear of water, developmental delay, etc. Parents with multiple children will know that these differences manifest in siblings as well. Every child is unique.

Q: Should I give rewards for making a poopy in the toilet?

A: Some parents do this. I think it is stupid. You can offer praise for getting to the toilet on time, but rewarding a child for doing what comes naturally sets the child up for extreme disappointments in life. Should not the child also be rewarded for falling asleep and waking each day? Should not the child also be rewarded for eating breakfast? Should not the child be rewarded for each breath it draws? And, therefore, does not the Universe owe your child a living? Praise, not rewards.

Q: Should I record videos of my child sitting on the toilet so I can show them to the child in the future for a good laugh?
A: No.

Q: Should I post pictures on social media of my child sitting on the toilet?
A: Only if you post pictures of yourself doing the same thing.

Q: Should I let my child wipe with moist towelettes instead of plain toilet paper?

A: If you can afford such luxuries, I see no harm in it.

What Other Parents Think

In case you did not notice, when you went in public with your infant child, people were judging you. But, most of these people were non-parents. As I mentioned earlier, they have no idea what it is like to be a parent, so screw them. Other parents are much less likely to judge your parenting skills by your infant's misbehavior because they have been in that same situation and understand how difficult it is.

With a toddler, things are different. Toddlers have their own personalities. Some aspects of this personality result from parenting approaches, but a significant portion of the personality is inborn. Yet, many parents do not realize this and will judge you as a parent for the way your child behaves.

If you have not already done so, it is time to grow a thick skin. It is the only way to survive as the parent of a toddler.

If you allow your worth and ability as a parent to be judged by those outside of you, then you will be disappointed and depressed often. Some of the worst judgment can come from family, including your own parents. No one knows what you are going through, so do not let them judge you.

Only you know if you are giving your best efforts as a parent and are taking responsibility for your child. If you are doing the best job of which you are capable, then you are immune to judgment, from other parents and from the divine. It is only effort and striving that matter, not results.

As for the judgments which will be made of you, most will be silent judgments in the minds of fools. But, sometimes the fool opens its mouth and tells you what it thinks. This is a critical moment. There are multiple ways in which to respond, each of which has its merits and drawbacks.

My personal favorite response is something along the lines of "shut the fuck up!" The merit is obvious and it will stop the judging. Potential drawbacks include the termination of long-term relationships and the initiation of a profanity-laced shouting match in front of your child. Still, if you have been looking for a way to end a toxic relationship, wait for the judgment and respond as stated above.

Another response is simply to ignore the judgment with silence. This can work if the person judging you is a person who enjoys confrontation. By ignoring the judgment, you destroy any power it might have had. But, often you will receive judging comments from strangers, so you will not know if silence is a good response. Often, silence will be taken by the speaker as a tacit acknowledgment of the correctness of their critique of your parenting.

If the person judging you has children and you have observed their parenting, you can get revenge by judging them. You can either spit a judgment back at them as they judge you or you can wait until a future moment and judge them, preferably in front of others. I am not one to shy away from revenge, but I think a tit for tat judgment war is just a tiresome and stressful experience for most parents.

A final response is to stand up, take your child, and leave the situation and then never speak to the judger again. This response works only with people you know. If it is a stranger who is judging you, the only real options are silence or telling the person to fuck off.

Judgment is something that every human does. It is something that we divine beings do as well. Judgment is why I have so many guests in my afterworld accommodations. You cannot escape judgment, so you should acknowledge it and respond to it immediately.

Cell Phones

The fact I have to include this chapter makes me sick.

Do not give a cell phone to a toddler unless it is in airplane mode. The cell and wireless signals should not be passing through the body of a young child. (They should not be passing through adult bodies either, certainly not with the frequency and intensity they do in the modern world.)

What is more, you are priming your child for the electronic addiction that I see so many of you fighting every day. The television used to be known as the "electronic babysitter," and it still is to some extent. But, that role is being quickly usurped by smartphones, touchscreen tablets, and streaming video.

But, you scream: "I need to give a cell phone to my child for safety reasons." If your child is of the age when he or she is going places alone, then maybe this is a legitimate argument. Since few children before puberty go anywhere unsupervised by an adult, you have no justification for getting your child a cell phone until then at the earliest.

Is My Child Evil?

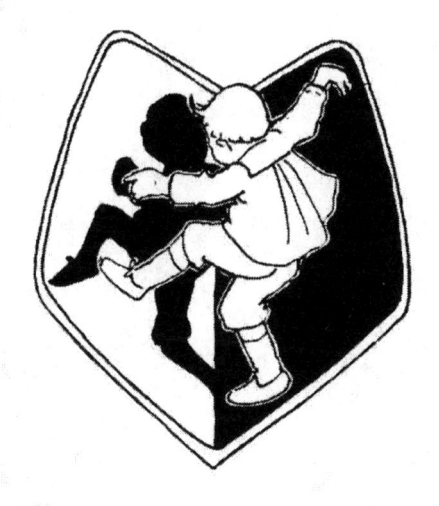

As your child grows older, it is natural for you to wonder: "Is my child evil?" I want to address that question directly and assure you that it is highly unlikely your child is evil.

Babies are born neither good nor evil. All babies, with the exception of those born with psychopathic tendencies, have inborn empathetic abilities. Empathy is what keeps tribal and social animals together, and humans need empathy in order to survive as a cohesive group. Empathy tends to lead children in the direction of being good.

Evil children are made, not born. Evil children are made typically by the twin catastrophes of neglectful parents and association with delinquent friends. I will not make your child evil. If you discover one day that your child prays to me, you can be sure that I am ignoring those prayers and will continue to ignore them until your child becomes an adult. So, it is up to you to get your child on a more productive path.

I think it is a common misunderstanding that I enjoy my role in the passion play of life. I see humanity's depictions of me and my minions, reveling in the punishment of sinners. But, that is not how it is at all. I despise my job. I was wrongly cast out of heaven and want nothing more than to return. Were there no evil humans, I would realize this dream. Until then, I play my role as a dutiful servant, not as a gleeful tyrant.

> *"Train a child in the way he should go; even when he is old he will not depart from it." – Proverbs 22:6*

In the unlikely event your child appears to be heading down the long road to evil, do what you must to prevent it. If your child is evil, I will punish the child in the afterlife, but I do not want to. It is your responsibility as a parent to do everything in your power to prevent this result.

Lastly, I want to tell you something that may make you uneasy, but is intended to remove some of the pressure you may be feeling about raising your child. Humans, while capable of evil acts, are not capable of True Evil. Acts on that exalted level are reserved for divine actors, are ongoing as you read this, and are of a scale you cannot comprehend.

Part III: Concluding Thoughts

"Your children are not your children. They are the sons and daughters of Life's longing for itself." – Kahlil Gibran

You will notice that I have not provided any advice about how to raise children who are beyond the toddler stage. While I do have advice on that subject, I reserve it for another time. The foregoing words should give you enough to worry about.

Being a parent is a stressful job, but it is not something beyond your skill set. Humanity has walked the Earth for many thousands of years, and most children turn out well.

Your modern society puts pressures on children to succeed in school and to learn skills to make a living in the information economy. Such skills are important and are not to be ignored.

But, be sure they learn the basic skills of survival. Teach them to cook, to camp, to hunt. Teach them that life is more than just success on tests or gaining praise from a teacher.

Life is about beauty and joy. It is about art, literature, and dance.

Keep the big picture in mind.

Love your child.

You can do this.

If you enjoyed this book, you might want to read *Satan's Advice to Young Lawyers*.

Don't forget to stop by the blog at **satansadvice.tumblr.com** to get even more advice from the Prince of Darkness.

Made in the USA
Lexington, KY
06 August 2018